T0129467

Cambridge Elements ≡

Elements of Improving Quality and Safety in Healthcare
edited by
Mary Dixon-Woods,* Katrina Brown,* Sonja Marjanovic,†
Tom Ling,† Ellen Perry,* and Graham Martin*
*THIS Institute (The Healthcare Improvement Studies Institute)
†RAND Europe

OPERATIONAL RESEARCH APPROACHES

Martin Utley, Sonya Crowe, and Christina Pagel

University College London

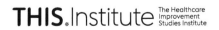
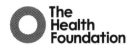

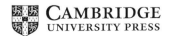

CAMBRIDGE
UNIVERSITY PRESS

University Printing House, Cambridge CB2 8BS, United Kingdom

One Liberty Plaza, 20th Floor, New York, NY 10006, USA

477 Williamstown Road, Port Melbourne, VIC 3207, Australia

314–321, 3rd Floor, Plot 3, Splendor Forum, Jasola District Centre,
New Delhi – 110025, India

103 Penang Road, #05–06/07, Visioncrest Commercial, Singapore 238467

Cambridge University Press is part of the University of Cambridge.

It furthers the University's mission by disseminating knowledge in the pursuit of
education, learning, and research at the highest international levels of excellence.

www.cambridge.org
Information on this title: www.cambridge.org/9781009236973
DOI: 10.1017/9781009236980

© THIS Institute 2022

This work is in copyright. It is subject to statutory exceptions
and to the provisions of relevant licensing agreements;
with the exception of the Creative Commons version the link for which is provided below,
no reproduction of any part of this work may take place without the written
permission of Cambridge University Press.

An online version of this work is published at doi.org/10.1017/9781009236980 under a Creative
Commons Open Access license CC-BY-NC-ND 4.0 which permits re-use, distribution and
reproduction in any medium for non-commercial purposes providing appropriate credit to the
original work is given. You may not distribute derivative works without permission. To view
a copy of this license, visit https://creativecommons.org/licenses/by-nc-nd/4.0

All versions of this work may contain content reproduced under license from third parties.

Permission to reproduce this third-party content must be obtained from these third-parties
directly.

When citing this work, please include a reference to the DOI 10.1017/9781009236980

First published 2022

A catalogue record for this publication is available from the British Library.

ISBN 978-1-009-23697-3 Paperback
ISSN 2754-2912 (online)
ISSN 2754-2904 (print)

Cambridge University Press has no responsibility for the persistence or accuracy of
URLs for external or third-party internet websites referred to in this publication
and does not guarantee that any content on such websites is, or will remain,
accurate or appropriate.

Every effort has been made in preparing this Element to provide accurate and up-to-date
information that is in accord with accepted standards and practice at the time of
publication. Although case histories are drawn from actual cases, every effort has been
made to disguise the identities of the individuals involved. Nevertheless, the authors,
editors, and publishers can make no warranties that the information contained herein is
totally free from error, not least because clinical standards are constantly changing through
research and regulation. The authors, editors, and publishers therefore disclaim all liability
for direct or consequential damages resulting from the use of material contained in this
Element. Readers are strongly advised to pay careful attention to information provided by
the manufacturer of any drugs or equipment that they plan to use.

Operational Research Approaches

Elements of Improving Quality and Safety in Healthcare

DOI: 10.1017/9781009236980
First published online: October 2022

Martin Utley, Sonya Crowe, and Christina Pagel
University College London

Author for correspondence: Martin Utley, m.utley@ucl.ac.uk

Abstract: Operational research is a collection of modelling techniques used to structure, analyse, and solve problems related to the design and operation of complex human systems. While many argue that operational research should play a key role in improving healthcare services, staff may be largely unaware of its potential applications. The authors explore operational research's wartime origins and introduce several approaches that operational researchers use to help healthcare organisations: address well-defined decision problems, account for multiple stakeholder perspectives, and describe how system performance may be impacted by changing the configuration or operation of services. The authors draw on examples that illustrate the valuable perspective that operational research brings to improvement initiatives and the challenges of implementing and scaling operational research solutions. The authors discuss how operational researchers are working to surmount these problems and suggest further research to help operational researchers have greater beneficial impact in healthcare improvement. This title is also available as Open Access on Cambridge Core.

Keywords: computer simulation modelling, heuristic search, multi-criteria decision analysis, operational research, location and allocation analysis

© THIS Institute 2022

ISBNs: 9781009236973 (PB), 9781009236980 (OC)
ISSNs: 2754-2912 (online), 2754-2904 (print)

Contents

1 Introduction

It is often argued that operational research, once branded 'the science of better', should play a key role in the analysis, design, and improvement of healthcare services.[1–3] But, despite some penetration into health systems, staff in many areas of health service planning, operation, and improvement may remain largely unaware of operational research and its potential applications.

In this Element, we first discuss the origins of operational research. We then give an overview of its application to improve healthcare services. Operational research comprises a wide range of methods and techniques and we do not attempt to cover them all here. Rather, we introduce some of the key concepts and common approaches before giving brief accounts of healthcare applications that demonstrate the range, potential, and, just as importantly, some of the limitations of the discipline. We also discuss some of the challenges of incorporating operational research into improvement initiatives and of working with operational researchers.

We focus predominantly on examples from the National Health Service (NHS) in the UK. And, where possible, we discuss work published in journals aimed at healthcare professionals or managers rather than examples published in technical journals targeted at other operational researchers.

2 What Is Operational Research?

In this section, we introduce definitions both of operational research and of the models that operational researchers construct when trying to solve problems. We also give an overview of the wartime origins of operational research. We then introduce a selection of the many different approaches that operational researchers may adopt when working to improve health services, before discussing some of the preparatory steps and behaviours common to these.

2.1 Operational Research as a Collection of Modelling Techniques

Operational research (referred to as operations research in the USA) can be viewed as a collection of conceptual, mathematical, statistical, and computational modelling techniques used for the structuring, analysis, and solving of problems related to the design and operation of complex human systems. These techniques range from approaches that systematically map the perspectives of individuals, professions, or organisations impacted by the problem being addressed, through to approaches for building and experimenting with a highly detailed mathematical or computational analogue of a healthcare service. A common element in these techniques is that the operational researcher, at some point in the course of their work, develops a 'model' of the system or problem.

The term model means different things to different people. Pidd gives the following definition for what operational researchers mean by a model in his excellent book *Tools for Thinking: Modelling in Management Science*:

> *A model is an external and explicit representation of part of reality as seen by the people who wish to use that model to understand, to change, to manage, and to control that part of reality.*[4]

We note that Pidd explicitly avoids the term 'improvement' in his definition, to acknowledge that an improvement from one perspective may constitute a worsening from another equally valid perspective. That said, many of the techniques introduced in this Element assume that the purpose of change is clear and agreed. As we will discuss, this can limit the acceptability of operational research techniques in some healthcare contexts.

Although a definition of operational research as a collection of certain modelling techniques works at one level, it is incomplete. The list of techniques deployed by operational researchers evolves over time and many people may use one or more of the techniques without identifying what they do as operational research. Indeed, the set of techniques used in operational research includes the theory of constraints and overlaps with those used in systems engineering, operations management, and industrial techniques such as Lean (see the Elements on systems mapping,[5] operations management approaches,[6] and Lean and associated techniques for process improvement[7]). To understand what binds the collection of techniques into a discipline, it is useful to cover the origins of operational research.

2.2 The Wartime Origins of Operational Research

Some of the techniques that comprise operational research were in use before the 1930s, for instance in the analysis of telecommunication networks and in the industrial time-and-motion studies of Taylor and others.[8] However, the term operational research was coined, and the discipline forged, immediately before and during the war effort of the Allied powers in the 1939–45 conflict of World War II.[9] Growing out of research related to the use of radar, academic scientists from different disciplines (including physicists, chemists, and geneticists) worked with the armed forces to frame and tackle the problems they faced, many of them related to the efficient deployment of resources. For example, one problem was to determine the optimal size of merchant convoys in the Atlantic Ocean that would minimise the losses of craft to submarine attacks given a fixed

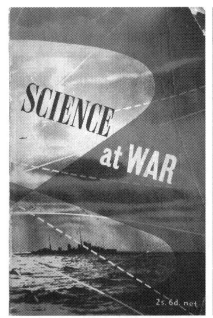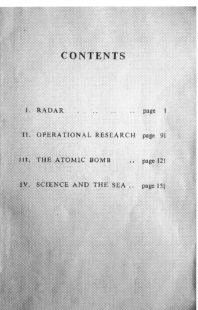

CONTENTS

Figure 1 Front cover and table of contents of the 1947 HMSO publication
Science at War,[9] showing the billing given to operational research
Cover design by Eileen Evans. Document held by The National Archives. Contains
public sector information licensed under the Open Government Licence v3.0.

availability of escort vessels. Another was how to increase the flying time of aircraft providing cover to convoys during attacks.

Figure 1 gives some indication of the importance attached to operational research at the end of the war, with the 1947 HMSO publication *Science at War*[9] giving as many pages to discussing operational research as it does to the atomic bomb.

2.3 Operational Research as More than a Collection of Techniques

Key to the success of operational research during the war was the acknowledgment by scientists that while they had expertise in data analysis and in using scientific methods to understand complex physical or biological systems, they did not understand warfare. To be useful, they needed to spend time listening to, learning from, and working alongside staff at all levels of the armed forces.

This was epitomised by Patrick Blackett, a professor of physics (and 1948 Nobel Prize winner) who served during the war as scientific adviser to the commander in chief of anti-aircraft command and as director of operational research for the admiralty. His wartime principles for effective operational research, reproduced by Royston,[10] included that it should be both:

- **collaborative**: 'An operational research section should be an integral part of a command and should work in the closest collaboration with the various departments at a command'
- **grounded**: 'All members of an operational research section should spend part of their time at operational stations in close touch with the personnel actually on the job'.

This recognition – that collaboration with workers at different levels of organisations and respecting their knowledge and experience are crucial – characterised the successful use of operational research across many industries in the postwar period, with large operational research groups formed within the coal and steel industries and in the railways.

In this sense, operational research is better defined as an ethos of problem framing and solving: applying scientific method and modelling techniques in collaboration with problem owners and subject experts to help understand and change the operation of complex organisations to some defined purpose. The textbook description of an operational researcher is someone who helps decision-makers frame their problem in a way amenable to systematic, rational analysis and then deploys the right tool for the job to solve the problem at hand. In reality, individual operational researchers rarely have proficiency across the whole spectrum of operational research approaches.

2.4 A Selection of Operational Research Approaches

In this section, we give a brief comparative account of several key approaches from the operational research toolkit, highlighting some of their applications in healthcare. For simplicity, we have grouped these into broad categories based on whether the primary intent of using the approach is to solve a well-defined decision problem with an agreed objective, to account for multiple perspectives on a problem, or to describe the behaviour of a system. We then discuss the use of combined approaches and the development of hybrid models.

2.4.1 Approaches for Solving Well-Defined Problems

First, we introduce the concept of optimisation. A frequently used example is the manufacture of cylindrical tin cans. Both the surface area and the volume of a cylinder can be calculated as functions of its height and the radius of the circular ends. Optimisation techniques can be used to identify for the manufacturer the single combination of height and radius that minimises the surface area of tin used to contain a given volume of soup (see Figure 2A).

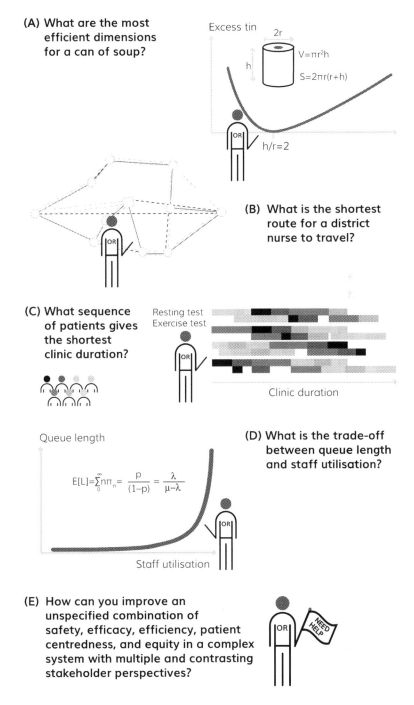

(A) What are the most efficient dimensions for a can of soup?

Excess tin

$V = \pi r^2 h$

$S = 2\pi r(r+h)$

$h/r = 2$

(B) What is the shortest route for a district nurse to travel?

(C) What sequence of patients gives the shortest clinic duration?

Resting test
Exercise test

Clinic duration

Queue length

$$E[L] = \sum_0^\infty n\pi_n = \frac{p}{(1-p)} = \frac{\lambda}{\mu-\lambda}$$

(D) What is the trade-off between queue length and staff utilisation?

Staff utilisation

(E) How can you improve an unspecified combination of safety, efficacy, efficiency, patient centredness, and equity in a complex system with multiple and contrasting stakeholder perspectives?

NEED HELP

Figure 2 Examples of problems amenable to operational research
OR = operational researcher

A key step in many of the approaches outlined in this Element is defining, for the sake of analysis, the purpose of the modelled system. This chimes with the focus of other improvement methods on defining what 'good' looks like and addressing the question: 'how will we know if we've made an improvement?' In operational research, this often involves writing down an 'objective function', which is a mathematical expression to quantify a key aspect of system performance. For a tin can, this is the equation expressing the surface area of the can in terms of its height and radius. In healthcare applications, this might be the distance travelled by a district nurse in terms of the order in which patients are visited (Figure 2B), or the duration of a clinic depending on the sequence of patients (Figure 2C).

Mathematical Programming

Mathematical programming is a group of optimisation techniques designed to identify how a system can be optimised by changing those features of a service considered to be under the control of decision-makers (called the design parameters or decision variables). A set of equations is constructed to relate the decision variables to the objective function and to other aspects of the system considered important (for instance, resource constraints or performance standards that must be met). A step-by-step process of calculation (called an algorithm) is deployed to identify a set of values for the decision variables that achieve the highest (or lowest) value for the objective while meeting the constraints. The algorithms used in mathematical programming are proven to work only for objective functions where the relationships between decision variables and objectives and constraints are relatively simple. Even then, they can be impractical for problems with a very large number of decision variables and constraints. Some problems in healthcare, while theoretically amenable to mathematical programming, would take many hours or even days or weeks of computer time to solve using these methods, which is too long if the problem needs to be solved on a daily basis. In such circumstances, researchers often turn to heuristic approaches, as described in the following paragraphs. For an overview of mathematical programming and other optimisation approaches applied in healthcare, see Crown et al.[11]

Heuristics and Heuristic Search

Heuristic approaches to problem-solving involve devising a set of rules to be applied, often iteratively, for obtaining acceptable solutions to problems, typically without any guarantee of finding an optimal solution. For the district nurse in Figure 2B, a simple heuristic would be to iteratively apply a rule of visiting the nearest patient they have not yet visited. Heuristic problem-solving has particular value in areas of scheduling and transportation and in staff rostering (see the discussion on nurse rostering in acute settings in Section 4.5).

Heuristic search is an alternative approach to improving the performance of a modelled system, in which a set of rules guides an iterative search of possible combinations of decision variables for a particular problem. Again the intent is to find a sufficiently good solution within acceptable computational time, without a guarantee that the solution is optimal.

2.4.2 Approaches to Account for Multiple Perspectives

Mathematical programming and heuristic search approaches assume, for the purposes of model building, that the objective of change is well-specified and agreed. This is often not the case, particularly in healthcare where patients, staff, and the management of different organisations within the system may take different views on the root of the problem being addressed, the desirability of different interventions, and the relative importance of different performance metrics.

Soft Systems Methodology

Problem-structuring methods are a group of operational research approaches that explicitly reject the notion of optimality in favour of identifying feasible courses of action that are acceptable to a group of stakeholders, while respecting that stakeholders will bring different values and value systems to the appraisal of alternatives.[12] For instance, patients, primary care clinicians, secondary care clinicians, and commissioners might all have different and valid perspectives on what constitutes a good quality healthcare service.

Soft systems methodology is one such approach that acknowledges and engages multiple perspectives.[13,14] It was developed to address complex multi-perspective issues through systematic learning about the problem and the relevant decision processes and mechanisms of change. Soft systems methodology involves developing a detailed account of the problematic situation motivating the desire for change, often in the form of a 'rich picture' depicting the people and organisations involved in a service, the issues as perceived from different perspectives, and the characteristics of potential improvements from a systems thinking perspective.

The researcher builds detailed conceptual models that articulate, in a systematic way, the different 'world views' (motivations, priorities, and constraints) of the different stakeholders. Through this process the researcher uses probing questions that identify feasible options for change and the likely impact of such changes. Augustsson et al. provide an overview of the application of soft systems methodology in healthcare.[15] Notable examples of UK works include efforts to improve postoperative services for infants with congenital heart disease that identified which patient groups to target with interventions such as home monitoring and multidisciplinary care teams,[16] and work at an acute hospital that identified simplifications in paperwork and a process for more frequent patient reviews which, when combined, reduced delays to discharge by 40%.[17]

Multi-Criteria Decision Analysis

Multi-criteria decision analysis is another set of operational research techniques designed to support decision-making in contexts where stakeholders may have markedly different perspectives on the relative value of different aspects of a system's performance. A quantitative model is built that links the characteristics of different options for change to the different metrics of performance that are of interest to the stakeholders.

One powerful strategy of multi-criteria decision analysis is to identify and discard options for change that are worse than others from at least one perspective and no better than others from any other perspectives. Other techniques within this approach are then used to build a shared understanding of the trade-offs between different perspectives, and to analyse individual and group preferences among options. Note that if there is no difference in opinion as to the relative importance of different criteria, multi-criteria decision analysis can simplify to a form of mathematical programming.

The application of multi-criteria decision analysis in healthcare is predominantly focused on questions of health policy or health technology assessment.[18,19] That said, example applications in the area of improvement include an exercise to support budgetary decisions in multi-agency initiatives to reduce teenage pregnancies in London, which suggested shifting investment from clinical services to other areas such as media campaigns and sex and relationship education,[20] and choosing between sites for a new health centre in the north of England based on assessments against seven weighted criteria, including the total cost, accessibility, and design of different options.[21] An example application in improving postnatal care is described in Section 4.4.

2.4.3 Approaches to Describe System Behaviour

The modelling approaches discussed in this section are intended primarily to offer a way of describing the behaviour of a system under a range of circumstances. These approaches are often used to determine and illustrate trade-offs between different aspects of system performance and to explore the likely impact of changes to the configuration or operation of a system.

Computer Simulation Modelling

The term simulation describes a wide range of research and training activities (further discussion can be found in the Element on simulation as an improvement technique[22]). Within operational research, simulation modelling involves constructing a model of the key components of a system. For instance, if simulating use of an emergency department, the components might be, for example, reception, triage, X-ray, minors and majors, along with the queues for each. The operation or behaviour of each component is specified by mathematical expressions or a set of rules, as are the relationships between components and the flows between components of patients, information, or other entities.

Simulation has wide application in healthcare.[23] In operational research, typically (but not exclusively), simulation is used when the nature of activities modelled at each component and the relationships between components are complex, such that the behaviour of the whole system over time and under different circumstances cannot be readily inferred from inspecting a set of equations. For instance, the time-dependent arrival patterns of patients to an emergency department, the subsequent prioritisation among evolving sets of patients based on clinical acuity, and the interplay between diagnostic processes, clinical decision-making, and how the flow of patients depends on the capacity available in other parts of the hospital cannot be modelled accurately without simulation. Learning about the system is instead generated by running the simulation on a computer and analysing the behaviour it exhibits, qualitatively or quantitatively, through the statistical analysis of model output. Features of the model corresponding to design parameters can then be changed (e.g. changing demand for services, or numbers of staff or beds) and the impact of these changes on model output can be analysed through experimentation.

Macro-simulation approaches, such as system dynamics, consider the high-level behaviour of a system and can be used to identify negative and positive feedback effects in complex healthcare systems. One example application is system-wide capacity planning for osteoarthritis in Alberta, Canada.[24] A review by Cassidy et al., written for a health services research audience, found that such approaches are often used to explore unintended consequences of proposed policies in urgent and emergency care and other highly connected systems[25] – for example, improvements designed for one target patient group having detrimental consequences for other users of the same service.

Micro-simulation approaches, such as discrete event simulation, operate at a patient level. Variables – such as the time between successive patients arriving, the duration and outcome of different clinical activities, and so on – are chosen at random from distributions on a patient-to-patient basis. The simulation model is then run hundreds or thousands of times for each experiment, sufficient for statistical analysis of the output from the model to generate meaningful insights. An example of computer simulation modelling to improve acute stroke care is discussed in Section 4.1.

Queueing Theory and Related Analytical Models of Patient Flow

Queueing theory is the mathematical analysis of how customers (or patients) flow through connected systems of processes (care activities) and the delays incurred as queues form and dissipate. The application of queueing theory involves using standard queueing equations, or deriving new ones to explore the performance of a system. Performance metrics include queue sizes, the waiting times experienced by different priority groups, the utilisation of resources, and the number of customers that baulk at the size of the queue or that join a queue but leave before being served. Applications in healthcare include capacity planning for specialist clinics,[26] understanding flows through mental health services,[27,28] and developing models to inform the staffing of accident and emergency services.[29]

Standard queueing equations are based on assumptions about how the time between the arrival of successive patients and the duration of care activities vary from patient to patient. For many real-world systems, these assumptions do not hold. This places some limitation on the validity of queueing theory results related to these systems, and perhaps a greater limitation on the acceptability of queueing theory to those working in the service. However, queueing theory remains a powerful tool to explore and communicate intrinsic trade-offs between different aspects of service performance due to day-to-day and patient-to-patient variability and uncertainty in terms of arrivals, treatment times, and lengths of stay (see Figure 2D).

2.4.4 Hybrid Models

In many operational research projects, the operational researcher uses more than one method, either through a comparative process of triangulation or with the output of one method feeding into another.[30] Hybrid models take this one step further, with one method embedded in another, or two computer implementations of operational research methods exchanging information iteratively in a combined run.[31] For example, a composite discrete event and system dynamic simulation model was used to look at the interaction between the operation of chlamydia screening clinics and the population-level dynamics of infection.[32]

2.5 Preparatory Steps to Modelling

As indicated, operational research comprises a wide range of approaches. The approach that an operational researcher might recommend for supporting a given improvement initiative depends on several factors. These include the nature of the service to be improved, the decisions and decision processes to be informed, the budget and time available for model development, and a degree of personal taste or comfort on the part of the operational researcher.

However, a unifying feature of operational research is that whatever modelling approach an operational researcher favours or chooses in a particular instance, a preparatory step in most operational research exercises is in-depth discussion of the problem as presented by clinicians and managers.[33,34] This typically involves site visits, shadowing and non-participant observation of relevant processes, and asking stupid and not-so-stupid questions. In our view this is an essential component of any high-quality piece of work. The operational researcher may wish to analyse exploratory data to check the self-diagnosis of the client organisation. This can often lead to useful insights for all parties. Indeed, sometimes a large proportion of the value added by an operational research exercise can be in this learning process and to have a problem studied from an operational researcher's perspective.

3 A Brief History of Operational Research in UK Healthcare

The Operational Research Club (the forerunner of the UK Operational Research Society) was founded in 1948, 3 months before the UK NHS, and operational researchers have attempted to inform the design and delivery of NHS services ever since. Relevant publications appeared in *The Lancet* as early as 1952.[35] In the following decades, operational research became an established academic discipline, with operational research groups in various domains of application formed within many UK universities. Not everyone has always agreed that healthcare services are a natural domain for applying quantitative operational research. For instance, Rosenhead set out in 1978 what he saw as fundamental problems with the reductionism of operational research when applied to a social system such as healthcare.[36]

Royston, a former president of the Operational Research Society, highlighted some of the successes in a 2008 paper to mark 50 years of operational research in health and healthcare.[10] In addition to input from academics, analysts working in the civil service for what is now the Department of Health and Social Care made important contributions. An operational research team was established in this department in the early 1970s, with the service later reconfigured to have operational researchers embedded in interdisciplinary teams, working in close collaboration with those specialising in policy development and delivery, which is the approach suggested by Blackett (see Section 2.3). These operational researchers informed ambulance response time standards when the NHS took on ambulance services in the late 1970s, funding allocation models and the design of screening programmes in the late 1980s, the design of NHS Direct in the late 1990s, and the setting of waiting time targets in the early 2000s.

The Operational Research and Evaluation unit of NHS England has worked on a number of projects, including the new models of care programme. Some regional NHS structures also include operational research groups, but they do not always survive the periodic reorganisation of regional and local NHS structures. Nine teams were disbanded with the abolition of the regional health authorities in the mid-1990s. Some primary care trusts were starting to develop some in-house operational research capability when they were abolished, and some clinical commissioning groups (for instance, NHS Bristol, North Somerset, and South Gloucestershire) and sustainable transformation partnerships (for instance, Kent and Medway) have an operational research or modelling function at the time of writing.

Development followed a similar trajectory in other countries with, for example, a Division of Operations Research established at the Johns Hopkins Hospital in Baltimore, USA, in 1956,[37] and operational research becoming a recognised academic discipline. Groups working in healthcare are active worldwide, with the programmes of European and US conferences giving a sense of the breadth of problems tackled.[38,39]

Today, healthcare operational research is seen as a subdiscipline within operational research, with dedicated streams at operational research conferences, health application editors within the major operational research journals, and specialist journals. The flavour of the work and the incentives at play differ from group to group, with some differences between groups situated in mathematics departments and those in management schools.

4 Operational Research in Action

In this section, we give illustrative examples of how some of the approaches discussed in Section 2.4 have been applied to improve the quality and safety of healthcare. Before doing so, we note that while operational research has undoubted potential to improve healthcare, a compelling body of empirical evidence to support its adoption is lacking. Evaluation of operational research projects is often limited to the feasibility and acceptability of the work (see for instance Glaize et al.[19]), rather than assessing the downstream impacts of decision-makers acting on the recommendations of a piece of operational research. Also, a large proportion of operational research projects do not influence decisions sufficiently for their recommendations to be empirically tested[23] and findings from individual operational research projects often are not adopted at scale.[40]

In partial explanation, the academic incentives at play in operational research promote the development of technically novel modelling approaches over empirical studies demonstrating their benefit,[41] with the hard work of implementation underestimated and undervalued.[42] In choosing examples, we have selected work that gives some account of implementation and a degree of evaluation. Even here, we acknowledge that operational research exercises have several of the characteristics of a complex intervention,[43] with the attendant problem of attributing any benefits observed to the operational research done as opposed to other factors.

4.1 Use of Simulation Modelling to Improve Acute Stroke Care

In 2010, a hospital in the south-west of England was concerned that too few of its new stroke patients were being treated with the thrombolytic drug alteplase.[44] At that time, alteplase was licensed for use only among patients who could be treated within 3 hours of onset of a confirmed ischaemic stroke. Within this 3-hour time window, a patient had to get to hospital, be identified as a likely stroke victim, and, crucially, have an MRI scan to rule out a haemorrhagic stroke (administering alteplase to a patient whose stroke is due to bleeding rather than to a clot would be catastrophic). The required time standard was met and thrombolysis administered in only 4% of stroke patients and the stroke team felt that the hospital could and should be doing better.

The acute stroke team worked with a team of operational researchers. Early discussions suggested that stroke patients were often caught up in congestion and delays within the hospital's emergency department, which generated some ideas for improvement. The operational research team built a discrete event simulation model to investigate the roots of the problem and estimate the likely impact of possible changes. They began by modelling the flows of acute stroke patients at the hospital up to and including the MRI scan and the commencement of any thrombolysis. Importantly, they converted the process measures (receipt of thrombolysis and time to thrombolysis) obtained through the simulation to a clinical measure of long-term disability outcome. In addition to these measures, they used the simulation to estimate the level of stroke team call-outs and high-priority MRI scans.

The simulation approach allowed the operational research team to account for time-of-day and day-of-week effects observed in emergency department processes and the availability of MRI scans. The simulation software generated animations of patient flow that facilitated feedback from clinicians on the completeness and accuracy of the workflows depicted. In discussion with the stroke team and a lead emergency department clinician, the operational research team used the simulation to explore the potential impact of having a triage clinician in the emergency department applying a screening tool to identify likely stroke patients, with the intention that likely candidates could then be referred directly to the stroke team, bypassing other processes in the emergency department. When other emergency department clinicians reviewed these analyses, they suggested that ambulance staff could also apply the screening tool and send a pre-alert for the stroke team to see the patient on arrival.

Using the simulation, researchers assessed the potential impact of these two interventions (screening followed by immediate stoke referral at triage in the emergency department, and screening by ambulance staff followed by pre-alert to the stroke team) alone and in combination with extending the time window for thrombolysis from 3 hours from stroke onset to 4.5 hours, as well as extending the eligibility criteria for thrombolysis to include people over 80 years old. The findings suggested that these changes could increase the level of thrombolysis treatment from 3% of all stroke patients other than existing inpatients (current practice) to 8.5% (screening and referral at emergency department triage), 10.4% (pre-alert from ambulance crew), or up to 22.8% (pre-alerts in combination with extending treatment time window and extending to the over-80s).

For many operational research studies, this is where the story would end. However, in this case, the hospital acted on the findings. They implemented stroke screening and referral at emergency department triage in December 2011, and worked with the local ambulance trust to introduce a stroke screening and pre-alert system in August 2012. Along the way, results from an international trial prompted the extension of thrombolysis to the over-80s.

The operational research team analysed process times and the proportion of stroke patients who were thrombolysed between January 2009 and August 2013. This analysis showed a 40% reduction in process times and an increase from 4.7% of all strokes thrombolysed in the period before the introduction of screening at emergency department triage to an average of 11.5% in the period after. Some of this increase was due to the extension of thrombolysis to the over-80s, but the increase of thrombolysis from 3.8% to 6.9% among patients under 80 whose stroke occurred outside the hospital showed the benefit of faster processes.[45]

The redesign of the acute stroke pathway at this hospital was a success, and the simulation modelling was important in allowing teams to safely experiment with different candidate interventions in silico and in providing a focus for discussions among the stroke team, physicians in the emergency department, and the ambulance trust. The simulation model was also valuable as a communication aid in explaining the work to other nearby trusts and led to similar exercises at four other hospitals.

4.2 Location of Urgent Care Centres

A recent example of location analysis in healthcare was the siting of urgent care centres in Cornwall, England.[46] The Sustainability and Transformation Partnership for Cornwall needed to provide urgent care while reducing demand at the county's emergency department. The partnership decided to establish urgent care centres in the county, but did not know how many to provide or where they should be sited.

The 13 locations in the county that already offered some form of urgent care were considered as candidate locations for a substantial urgent care centre. The partnership judged one of these candidates to be an obvious choice because of the existing services at that site. They also acknowledged that some Cornish residents would use urgent care providers in their neighbouring county.

The operational researcher working with the partnership used a form of location–allocation optimisation analysis to inform these decisions. Using 3 years' worth of data on the home postcode of patients receiving urgent care, they built a computer model that allowed evaluation of any proposed configuration of urgent care centres. A configuration was defined by choosing how many and which of 12 sites to use alongside the one obvious choice and three centres in the bordering county. Each configuration was evaluated on the weighted mean travel time between the centre of postcode districts in the county and the nearest urgent care centre under that configuration. The contribution from each postcode was weighted by the historic demand for urgent care among patients resident in that postcode.

By evaluating every possible configuration, the researcher identified the relationship between the number of urgent care centres and average travel times, and was able to identify the best combination of sites if a fixed number were chosen. Informed by this analysis, the partnership chose to establish three urgent care centres in the county and sited them at the locations identified by the model. The analysis predicts a patient will travel on average for 19 minutes. This analysis includes caveats, notably an assumption that patient journeys start from the home address, but it was a systematic way for decision-makers to explore one important facet of this facility location problem.

The analysis was facilitated by the limited number – 4,096 – of possible configurations of urgent care centres in Cornwall, making it feasible to evaluate each one. For larger-scale problems, this isn't the case. King et al. explored the location of specialist paediatric intensive care retrieval teams in England and Wales, choosing between 8 and 12 locations from a possible 35.[47] This corresponds to over 1.5 billion possible configurations. In such cases, optimisation and heuristic search techniques of operational research are computationally efficient ways to find very good or optimal combinations of location. Using open-source libraries of optimisation routines, the authors established that 55% of patients could be reached by a retrieval team within 90 minutes and 98% of patients could be reached by a retrieval team within 3 hours (travelling by road). But they also found that if the current time-to-bedside standard of 3 hours was tightened, the service would struggle to meet it without expanding the use of aircraft and/or increasing the number of retrieval team locations. They identified that the optimal location of 11 teams could increase the percentage of patients likely to be reached within 90 minutes from 55% under the current configuration to 70%. Their analysis was deliberately simplistic, providing a preliminary exploration of the potential room for improvement in any reconfiguration of services, but illustrates the value that operational research could bring to an ongoing national review of paediatric intensive care and retrieval.

4.3 Organising Home Care in Sweden

Delivering care in people's own homes presents tough organisational problems.

- Providers face demand for visits to patients that are potentially subject to constraints on when the visit should happen, and to the minimum set of qualifications required of the staff member for the activities planned.
- The total number of staff available is limited, as is the availability of individual staff members within the planning period.
- The number of individuals to visit a patient over the duration of their care should be as low as possible, both for continuity of care and so that patients are not exposed to too many different people.
- The care required can change at short notice.
- Regulations limit the total number of hours that individuals can work and further stipulate the number and durations of breaks they are permitted.
- Different members of staff have different preferred modes of transport.
- Allocation of workload across staff should be as fair as possible.
- In some settings, staff need to start and finish their working day at a base unit.

Planners are routinely tasked with constructing staff visit schedules and routes that satisfy these demands within the constraints and avoid excessive travelling time for staff. In many organisations in the UK and elsewhere, this job is left for senior nurses to do manually, with information technology used only to provide information and to check and record solutions. Finding a workable solution, let alone a good one, is very time-consuming and cognitively very challenging.

In 2001, local authority care providers in Danderyd, Sweden, worked with a software company to build an operational research-based tool to address the combination of staff-to-patient allocation, staff scheduling, and staff routing problems. The resulting system, Laps Care, has since been adopted by over 200 providers across 50 municipalities in Sweden.[48]

The operational research algorithm at the heart of Laps Care is an example of heuristic search. A key consideration for the developers was to limit the time taken by the software to return a solution to 5–10 minutes, to facilitate repeated use on a daily basis. The first step in the process is to assign every visit to a different staff member, with all of these staff members given a route that visits just one patient. This inefficient starting set of staff routes is then reduced by iteratively amalgamating routes, finding the best combinations at each iteration (in terms of route duration and compatibility with patient time windows and staff competencies), and then testing the new set of routes against the current best set. If no improvement is found, the algorithm either stops or (if sufficient computational time remains) takes some of the routes from the current best set, breaks them up, and restarts the amalgamation process. This approach finds good solutions in less time than taken by staff performing the job manually. The system increases the number of patient visits per member of staff per hour by 5–15% and reduces the time spent by staff on constructing schedules by around a third. Across the customer base of Laps Care, these and other indirect benefits have been estimated to have a monetary value of around €100 million.[48]

Some of the algorithms deployed in Laps Care are very sophisticated (our description is simplified). However, especially striking is the careful iterative design work, both in building the interface around the algorithms and in ensuring the appropriateness of the information feeding the algorithms. For example, the map tools that form the basis of the routing came from the automotive industry and the developers manually adjusted maps to account for routes open to workers on foot or bicycle that were not open to those driving.

4.4 Shaping Postnatal Care Improvement Using Multi-Criteria Decision Support

The postnatal care pathway for mothers and newborns in the UK is delivered in acute hospitals, the mother's home, and in community clinics. Isolated quality improvements may be possible within each setting, but differences in the priority attached to different aspects of quality may mean that isolated initiatives are misaligned. Crucially, changes in one part of the pathway can require additional resource that may not be available without reducing the resource invested elsewhere in the pathway.

Operational researchers worked closely with nursing and midwifery researchers to develop a tool to support improvement initiatives in postnatal care.[49] The resulting Postnatal Resource Allocation Model (PRAM) explores the impact of altering resource allocation across the postnatal care pathway. To develop PRAM, researchers used a mix of qualitative methods to understand the current operation of services and different stakeholder perspectives on quality in postnatal care. They collated a knowledge base from the literature, augmented by case studies and expert opinion. These fed into the development and use of a quantitative modelling framework that incorporated explicit assumptions about the links between changes in resource allocation and changes in quality.

Conceptions of quality within healthcare are essential to this form of analysis and are highly contested (see the Element on values and ethics[50]). In this instance, the team mapped aspects of postnatal care to the internationally recognised quality domains of safety, effectiveness, timeliness, equity, and the extent to which care is recipient-centred.[51]

The inputs for PRAM are the amount of resource devoted to particular activities (for instance, staffing of the postnatal ward, the typical length of stay on the postnatal ward, and the number of home visits made by a midwife following discharge). Outputs are numeric values for the anticipated quality of the service under that scenario of resource allocation. A prediction of quality for a scenario is calculated separately for each quality domain and in aggregate for each of four groups of new mothers who have ascending levels of medical, mental health, and social need.

The equations to predict quality assume that each measure of quality increases proportionally with resource input up to a maximum level, beyond which no further improvement is possible. A separate equation is used for each pairing of design parameter and domain of quality. In developing the model, each of these equations has to be calibrated. Additionally, each domain is given a weighting, which is used in calculating aggregate quality scores. To calibrate the model, the research team reviewed the literature on quality in postnatal care, filling gaps in the scientific evidence base using expert opinion and/or data and knowledge gathered outside research. The PRAM tool includes a facility for users to explore and question the sources used, which are categorised by relevance and rigour.

One service in the north of England used PRAM to inform changes to their postnatal service. The team validated PRAM by using it to assess the current allocation of resources, then checking through discussions with staff that the deficits in quality highlighted by the PRAM analysis were consistent with their perceptions of the service. The research team then used PRAM to explore with staff the potential impact of several scenarios for revised allocation of resources. One scenario entailed: earlier discharge from the postnatal ward; a net reduction in staffing, but an increase in feeding support on the ward; additional home visits for higher need groups; and an additional feeding and parenting support clinic for all groups. This scenario was anticipated to reduce total costs by 7% and to improve quality for all groups, with marked improvements among higher need groups.

An ongoing process evaluation found that the use of PRAM had increased participation of staff in the redesign process compared with previous improvement initiatives, had acted as a useful focus for sharing knowledge and service data between stakeholders, and led to increased understanding of current services and the perspectives of different stakeholders on options for change.[49]

4.5 Nurse Rostering in Acute Settings

We described in Section 4.3 the use of operational research methods to schedule staff activities in home-based care in Sweden. A related problem in acute settings involves determining which nurses will work which shifts. The roster for a ward needs to ensure adequate staffing (in terms of the numbers and competencies of staff members) and a degree of fairness across staff while meeting regulatory constraints on shift durations and working patterns. Rosters should account for requested leave, be robust to staff sickness, and perhaps be able to take into account individual staff preferences.

Many approaches have been developed to tackle this problem.[52] Formulations go well beyond the criteria given in the last paragraph, including work from Kuwait on incorporating any need for administering the last rites by ensuring that adherents of dominant religions are represented among the nurses on duty.[53] The problem is typically framed as a mathematical programming problem. The decision variables indicate whether each member of staff is scheduled for each shift. Hard constraints (those that have to be met by solutions) enforce stipulated staffing requirements, working patterns, and account for staff availability and other essential features. The objective function is typically a weighted function of the salary costs of a solution and the extent to which a solution breaches soft constraints such as staff preferences. The developers of new algorithms can use test cases to benchmark their approach against approaches proposed by other researchers. Adequate solutions to this technically complex rostering problem can be obtained in a matter of minutes on a standard PC. But poor take-up of this kind of operational research approach is the norm in healthcare, where staff still spend many hours each month constructing rosters manually – an arduous, cognitively difficult, and usually thankless task of combinatorial optimisation seen as a rite-of-passage by senior staff but rarely covered in the syllabus of nursing degrees.[54] In our own work, we have seen talented senior nurses struggle to construct rosters using software that offers no help, and working with information on staff availability recorded on spreadsheets and post-it notes, or even a napkin.

The poor penetration of operational research approaches for staff rostering in healthcare practice has prompted its own literature. A survey of the authors of academic nurse rostering optimisation models found that only 30% of models had been implemented by hospitals, with many of these limited to single sites. Some authors openly admitted that they had developed their approach with no explicit intent for their work to be implemented. Where academic models were implemented at some scale, there was little focus in the literature on sharing and learning the lessons from successful implementation.[55] Surveying the approaches to rostering in US hospitals highlighted that the dominant software systems with a nurse-scheduling function do not take an optimisation approach and that standalone optimisation approaches to narrowly defined problems are not attractive commercially.[55]

A mixed-methods analysis of rostering practice and roster quality in Malaysia suggests other reasons for the poor uptake of operational research rostering methods.[54] A key point is that many of the criteria for a roster viewed in the literature as hard constraints are often violated in practice, and so are not truly hard constraints. Also, many of the considerations that influence the construction of rosters in practice are absent from model formulations. Rostering was found in this study be to a highly political exercise with planners aiming to balance the technical merits of the roster with tacit considerations, including power dynamics, granting favours, and avoiding conflict.

From this perspective, we argue that operational researchers need to avoid a narrow gaze that only sees the technical complexity of problems and not the social complexity. If clinicians and managers are struggling with a technically complex operational problem, the researcher should not assume that it is the technical complexity alone that causes the difficulty.

5 Critiques of the Approach

In this section, we set out our view of the strengths and challenges of working with operational researchers and operational research models.

5.1 Strengths of Operational Research

The systematic and disciplined construction of explicit models (quantitative or qualitative) that relate aspects of system performance to those elements of a system that people feel they control offers several advantages.

First, operational research models can reveal and quantify relationships between different aspects of system performance, including trade-offs among different aspects of performance that are considered beneficial for organisations, staff, or patients. Second, such models can help place realistic expectations on the scale of impact on different aspects of performance that is achievable.

Operational research analyses can be used to screen ideas for which aspects of a service to alter, or to identify and target improvement initiatives on those changes that are likely to have the most beneficial impact.[41] In the example discussed in Section 4.1 about improving acute stroke care, the team explored and discarded several interventions as being unlikely to lead to a marked improvement before settling on those that were seriously considered for implementation. Operational research also offers a range of approaches that can help organisations to place relative values on the different aspects of system performance that may be changed through improvement initiatives.

Finally, for circumstances where an explicit goal can be framed, operational research provides a set of sophisticated algorithms for identifying the changes to a system likely to give the biggest improvement. This means that operational research can add value to other improvement methods that focus only on generating ideas for change, or on helping organisations implement change, or on the empirical evaluation of changes as they are implemented.

5.2 Challenges of Operational Research

5.2.1 Operational Research May Offer a Naïve World View

While quantitative operational research techniques can bring great value to improvement initiatives, they are intrinsically reductionist. Even the qualitative techniques of soft operational research cannot capture the full complexity of healthcare or the full nuance of different stakeholder perspectives. This can be a weakness, particularly for quantitative models that focus on optimisation. The concept of the objective function, introduced in Section 2.4, implicitly assumes model completeness, requiring that the purpose of the system can be expressed mathematically using only variables contained within the model. Perhaps more importantly, the concept of the objective function presupposes that the purpose of a system is, or can be made, explicit, and is or can be agreed by the people responsible for the design and operation of that system.

If the notion of explicit and agreed objectives within healthcare is somewhat naïve, the operational researchers' view of decision-making processes may sometimes be outright fanciful when applied in a healthcare context. The origins of operational research in serving organisations with clear command and control structures are important here. Healthcare has a more complex system of power structures within and between professions. Much of the operational research literature discusses the 'decision-maker' as if this were an individual with agency to change at will the design parameters in the modelled system. This world view is not consistent with the social and political processes through which change is enacted in healthcare.

Furthermore, when working closely with organisations, the explicit nature of operational research models can present difficulties. In politically hot contexts, some within organisations may be reluctant to formally acknowledge the trade-offs between different aspects of performance that intrinsically limit how well a service can perform. For example, in the nurse rostering problem discussed in Section 4.5, organisations in practice may occasionally allow a level of staffing on a ward that is lower than what is considered safe, but they can be reluctant to acknowledge the near-inevitability of such breaches in the black-and-white of a model formulation.

One response might be for operational researchers to limit their work to aspects of healthcare where the problems are technically complex but socially and politically simple. But a more ambitious approach might involve operational researchers seeking to understand more fully the tensions between different perspectives and how change is typically brought about in the organisation they are working with. Armed with this kind of insight, they may be better enabled to design models and ways of presenting and talking about model output that strengthen improvement initiatives. Working without that close engagement risks fundamentally misconceiving the problem and the decision processes the researcher aims to inform.

In short, while reductionist models provide a simplified view of healthcare, their use can still be beneficial. Model developers must work to understand the elements of reality that are not included in the model and communicate the inevitable caveats that this reductionism brings to interpreting the model output within decision processes. The growing field of behavioural operational research seeks to address some of these problems by including behavioural factors within models (arguably making models less reductive) and by studying how the behaviour of operational researchers and other actors through the research process affects the uptake and impact of operational research.[56]

A related weakness of operational research approaches is the low level of patient and public involvement in the development of operational research interventions. Patient and public perspectives are captured in problem-structuring methods such as soft systems methodology, and the original proponents of these methods envisaged them being used in a way that would today be labelled as co-production. However, operational researchers have only recently started to look for ways of involving patients and the public in the process of model building and experimentation.[57] Further discussion of co-production can be found in the Element on co-producing and co-designing.[58]

5.2.2 Operational Research May Offer Bespoke Solutions for an Off-the-Peg World

Many operational research models are built to be generic, such that they can be configured to describe many different instances of the same problem. For example, in the stroke work, this means being able to vary patient arrival rates, MRI access, and stroke team staffing to match the situation in a different hospital.[45] However, much of the value of operational research lies in the modelling process rather than in the models and solutions developed, and the shared understanding built through the modelling process cannot be easily replicated in new settings without a commitment of time and effort from both the operational research team and the new organisation. This has implications for the scaling of operational research interventions. For instance, the team that did the stroke work faced new challenges when spreading the work to different hospitals.

Two of the examples of successful applications that we discussed in Section 4 come from an operational research group in the south-west of England. This group has been active in supporting local improvement initiatives for over a decade, accompanying this with a programme of awareness raising, education, and training on operational research modelling approaches. Without this groundwork and relationship building, it is likely that modelling exercises would have had less impact. Sustained personal relationships and trust between operational researchers and host organisations have been important to the success of our own work,[33] with these formalised through modellers in residence[33,59] and embedded researcher roles,[60] and interdisciplinary embedded research teams.[61]

5.2.3 Operational Research Solutions Create Problems at Implementation

One of the advantages of operational research models is that they can explore the implications of changing several aspects of a service in combination. Because of this, operational research methods can find that the biggest improvements to service performance may come from major changes to how a system is configured or operated. This makes some operational research solutions incompatible with some improvement methods that are rooted in testing small incremental changes. Additionally, while the running costs of the current configuration and any alternatives explored tend to be accounted for in operational research models, they rarely account for the one-off costs and other practical consequences of major change. For example, the model used to assess different combinations of location for paediatric intensive care transport services did not incorporate explicitly the one-off costs of removing some services and establishing others.[47]

Many operational research methods are implemented through software tools, and operational research projects often require the development of software to implement a solution, typically by a developer. To use the software in the longer term, an organisation must support its maintenance and use by healthcare staff, and the software must be integrated, or at least be compatible with the organisation's existing IT products. This can be achieved, but operational researchers rarely have the skills to build software to professional standards or the incentives or inclination to provide user support. Note that the development of Laps Care discussed in Section 4.3 involved a software company from the start. In this example, few academics would see value in altering digital maps to account for cycle routes and pedestrian-only routes, despite this mundane sort of work being recognised as important to success.

There is a broader point also. Just as operational researchers do not necessarily have the software design and development skills to produce user-friendly implementations of their models, they may not necessarily have the soft skills required to communicate effectively with and influence the healthcare service staff who are key to the decision processes they seek to inform. One approach has been to base operational researchers alongside an improvement team whose members do have those skills.[62]

5.3 Finding and Working with Operational Researchers

As discussed in Section 5.2.2, the need for a bespoke (or at least made to measure) modelling process limits the extent to which operational research solutions can readily be translated from one organisation to another. It also raises the question of whether there are enough operational researchers working in healthcare to serve the needs of improvement in the NHS. While some parts of the UK are particularly well served by modelling teams, notably Wales and the south-west of England, others are less so.

Finding good operational researchers can be difficult. A directory of operational research academics and modelling practitioners interested and/or active in healthcare is available online.[63] Those looking to engage with an operational research team should reasonably expect that they:

- show a genuine interest in the service to be improved, wanting to meet on site and shadow or observe processes in action
- ask questions that probe and challenge the objectives of the improvement initiative, potentially to a slightly annoying extent
- present a number of ideas on potential approaches and how this choice might be influenced by the nature of the decision processes within the organisation, data availability, and resource considerations.

While an operational researcher should rightly be interested in the details of how services work, be wary of complexity fetishism. Some modellers like building complex models, and people working in healthcare often like to be told how complex their problems are. If indulged too much, this tendency can encourage very large, very complex models that give a good description of the status quo but are unwieldy when wanting to study the potential impact of change.

6 Conclusions

The logistical problems that have drawn operational researchers to work in healthcare for decades remain and are likely to increase as pressure on resources increases. In this Element, we have discussed a range of operational research approaches and given example applications in healthcare that show the benefits that operational researchers, their models, and their algorithms can bring to improvement initiatives. We have considered some of the limitations to the discipline and how these are being addressed through methodological developments and new ways of building partnerships between operational researchers, NHS organisations, and other improvement disciplines.

The examples we give of operational research in action demonstrate the breadth of its capability and the fact that operational research is informing important decisions related to the improvement of healthcare services across sectors. As we have discussed, often the benefits of operational research come from the construction of a model that allows the likely impact of change to be assessed. However, we have also seen that to build these models it is necessary to leave out some aspects of reality and simplify others, and that this reductionism can limit the perceived validity of operational research approaches among clinicians and managers. It can also lead operational researchers to take a simplified view of how decisions are made in healthcare. To remedy this, we encourage the growing trend of incorporating operational research approaches within wider improvement initiatives that engage fully with the complexities of realising change within and across healthcare organisations. We are also supportive of other efforts to close the gap between operational researchers and healthcare organisations by enhancing the awareness of modelling and modelling capabilities of the analytical workforce within healthcare.

While there is technical research to be done *within* operational research on how best to connect operational research modelling to the growing field of analytics and data science in healthcare, and there will always be research on finding better algorithms, there is a stronger need for research *about* operational research. In particular, a greater focus is required on building an empirical evidence base for the adoption of operational research approaches to improvement in healthcare. We lack comprehensive research that characterises and quantifies the costs and benefits of developing, implementing, and scaling operational research solutions. It would also be valuable to grow an evidence base on the different behaviours and collaborative approaches that operational researchers adopt when working with healthcare organisations, to establish approaches to the conduct of operational research that facilitate successful implementation of operational research models.

In summary, for the technically, socially, and politically complex problems often faced in improvement practice, operational research will rarely provide a complete solution, but will almost always bring a fresh perspective and can, at its best, make some very valuable contributions.

7 Further Reading

- Hulshof et al.[64] – a wide-ranging review of operational research approaches in healthcare.
- For those interested in the wartime origins of operational research and its development in the following decades, see Kirby.[65]
- Royston[10] – a brief history of the application of operational research to problems in health and healthcare.

- Pidd[4] – a broader account of operational research modelling, which goes beyond healthcare and spans the quantitative approaches focused on in this Element and the more qualitative approaches of problem-structuring methods.
- Winston and Goldberg[66] – a rigorous introduction to the key concepts and algorithms of quantitative operational research approaches.

Contributors

Martin Utley wrote first draft with contributions on scope, structure, and content from Sonya Crowe and Christina Pagel. All authors have approved the final version.

Conflicts of Interest

None.

Acknowledgements

We thank the peer reviewers and editors for their insightful comments and recommendations to improve the Element. A list of peer reviewers is published at www.cambridge.org/IQ-peer-reviewers.

Funding

This Element was funded by THIS Institute (The Healthcare Improvement Studies Institute, www.thisinstitute.cam.ac.uk). THIS Institute is strengthening the evidence base for improving the quality and safety of healthcare. THIS Institute is supported by a grant to the University of Cambridge from the Health Foundation – an independent charity committed to bringing about better health and healthcare for people in the UK.

About the Authors

Martin Utley is Professor of Operational Research in the Clinical Operational Research Unit at University College London, where he works to assist those planning, delivering, or evaluating health services by developing, adapting, and applying operational research techniques.

Sonya Crowe is Professor of Operational Research and Director of the Clinical Operational Research Unit at University College London. She has made key contributions to operational research applied to health protection policy and currently leads work spanning clinical outcomes, service delivery, and innovation in health and social care.

Christina Pagel is Professor of Operational Research in the Clinical Operational Research Unit at University College London. She currently leads work on paediatric intensive care and congenital heart surgery. She is passionate about the analysis and communication of data to help improve public health and healthcare delivery.

Creative Commons Licence

The online version of this work is published under a Creative Commons licence called CC-BY-NC-ND 4.0 (https://creativecommons.org/licenses/by-nc-nd/4.0). It means that you're free to reuse this work. In fact, we encourage it. We just ask that you acknowledge THIS Institute as the creator, you don't distribute a modified version without our permission, and you don't sell it or use it for any activity that generates revenue without our permission. Ultimately, we want our work to have impact. So if you've got a use in mind but you're not sure it's allowed, just ask us at enquiries@thisinstitute.cam.ac.uk.

The printed version is subject to statutory exceptions and to the provisions of relevant licensing agreements, so you will need written permission from Cambridge University Press to reproduce any part of it.

All versions of this work may contain content reproduced under licence from third parties. You must obtain permission to reproduce this content from these third parties directly.

References

1. Buhaug H. Long waiting lists in hospitals: operational research needs to be used more often and may provide Answers. *BMJ* 2002; 324: 252–3. https://doi.org/10.1136/bmj.324.7332.252.

2. Young T, Brailsford S, Connell C, et al. Using industrial processes to improve patient care. *BMJ* 2004; 328: 162–4. https://doi.org/10.1136/bmj.328.7432.162.

3. Pitt M, Dodds S, Bensley D, Royston G, Stein K. The potential for operational research. *Br J Healthc Manag* 2009; 15: 22–7. https://doi.org/10.12968/bjhc.2009.15.1.37894.

4. Pidd M. *Tools for Thinking: Modelling in Management Science, 2nd ed.* Chichester: John Wiley and Sons; 2002.

5. Komashie A, Kotiadis K, Lamé G, Clarkson PJ. Systems mapping. In: Dixon-Woods M, Brown K, Marjanovic S, et al., editors. *Elements of Improving Quality and Safety in Healthcare.* Cambridge: Cambridge University Press; forthcoming.

6. Lewis MA, Vasilakis C. Operations management approaches. In: Dixon-Woods M, Brown K, Marjanovic S, et al., editors. *Elements of Improving Quality and Safety in Healthcare.* Cambridge: Cambridge University Press; forthcoming.

7. Radnor Z, Williams S. Lean and associated techniques for process improvement. In: Dixon-Woods M, Brown K, Marjanovic S, et al., editors. *Elements of Improving Quality and Safety in Healthcare.* Cambridge: Cambridge University Press; forthcoming.

8. Clark GW. Machine-shop engineering roots of Taylorism: the efficiency of machine-tools and machinists, 1865–1884. In: Spender J-C, Kijne HJ, editors. *Scientific Management: Frederick Winslow Taylor's Gift to the World?* Boston, MA: Springer; 1996: 33–62. https://doi.org/10.1007/978-1-4613-1421-9_2.

9. Crowther J, Whiddington R. *Science at War.* London: HMSO; 1947.

10. Royston G. One hundred years of operational research in health – UK 1948–2048. *J Oper Res Soc* 2009; 60(suppl1): S169–79. https://doi.org/10.1057/jors.2009.14.

11. Crown W, Buyukkaramikli N, Thokala P, et al. Constrained optimization methods in health services research – an introduction: report 1 of the ISPOR Optimization Methods Emerging Good Practices Task Force. *Value Health* 2017; 20: 310–9. https://doi.org/10.1016/j.jval.2017.01.013.

12. Smith CM, Shaw D. The characteristics of problem structuring methods: a literature review. *Eur J Oper Res* 2019; 274: 403–16. https://doi.org/10 .1016/j.ejor.2018.05.003.

13. Checkland P. Soft systems methodology: a thirty year retrospective. *Syst Res Behav Sci* 2000; 17: S11–S58. https://doi.org/10.1002/1099-1743 (200011)17:1+<::AID-SRES374>3.0.CO;2-O.

14. Checkland P, Poulter J. Soft systems methodology. In: Reynolds M, Holwell S, editors. *Systems Approaches to Managing Change: A Practical Guide*. London: Springer; 2010: 191–242. https://doi.org/10.1007/978-1-84882-809-4_5.

15. Augustsson H, Churruca K, Braithwaite J. Re-energising the way we manage change in healthcare: the case for soft systems methodology and its application to evidence-based practice. *BMC Health Serv Res* 2019; 19: 666. https://doi.org/10.1186/s12913-019-4508-0.

16. Crowe S, Brown K, Tregay J, et al. Combining qualitative and quantitative operational research methods to inform quality improvement in pathways that span multiple settings. *BMJ Qual Saf* 2017; 26: 641–52. http://dx .doi.org/10.1136/bmjqs-2016-005636.

17. Emes M, Smith S, Ward S, Smith A. Improving the patient discharge process: implementing actions derived from a soft systems methodology study. *Health Syst* 2019; 8: 117–33. https://doi.org/10.1080/20476965 .2018.1524405.

18. Hansen P, Devlin N. Multi-criteria decision analysis (MCDA) in healthcare decision-making. *Oxf Res Encycl Econ Finance* 2019. https://doi.org/10 .1093/acrefore/9780190625979.013.98.

19. Glaize A, Duenas A, Martinelly CD, Fagnot I. Healthcare decision-making applications using multicriteria decision analysis: a scoping review. *J Multi-Criteria Decis Anal* 2019; 26: 62–83. https://doi.org/10.1002/mcda .1659.

20. Franco LA, Lord E. Understanding multi-methodology: evaluating the perceived impact of mixing methods for group budgetary decisions. *Omega* 2011; 39: 362–72. https://doi.org/10.1016/j.omega.2010.06.008.

21. Dehe B, Bamford D. Development, test and comparison of two multiple criteria decision analysis (MCDA) models: a case of healthcare infrastructure location. *Expert Syst Appl* 2015; 42: 6717–27. https://doi.org/10.1016/j .eswa.2015.04.059.

22. Brazil V, Purdy E, Bajaj K. Simulation as an improvement technique. In: Dixon-Woods M, Brown K, Marjanovic S, et al., editors. *Elements of Improving Quality and Safety in Healthcare*. Cambridge: Cambridge University Press; forthcoming.

23. Brailsford SC, Harper PR, Patel B, Pitt M. An analysis of the academic literature on simulation and modelling in health care. *J Simul* 2009; 3: 130–40. https://doi.org/10.1057/jos.2009.10.

24. Vanderby SA, Carter MW, Noseworthy T, Marshall DA. Modelling the complete continuum of care using system dynamics: the case of osteo-arthritis in Alberta. *J Simul* 2015; 9: 156–69. https://doi.org/10.1057/jos.2014.43.

25. Cassidy R, Singh NS, Schiratti P-R, et al. Mathematical modelling for health systems research: a systematic review of system dynamics and agent-based models. *BMC Health Serv Res* 2019; 19: 845. https://doi.org/10.1186/s12913-019-4627-7.

26. Izady N. Appointment capacity planning in specialty clinics: a queueing approach. *Oper Res* 2015; 63: 916–30. https://doi.org/10.1287/opre.2015.1391.

27. Koizumi N, Kuno E, Smith TE. Modeling patient flows using a queuing network with blocking. *Health Care Manag Sci* 2005; 8: 49–60. https://doi.org/10.1007/s10729-005-5216-3.

28. Utley M, Gallivan S, Pagel C, Richards D. Analytical methods for calculating the distribution of the occupancy of each state within a multi-state flow system. *IMA J Manag Math* 2009; 20: 345–55. https://doi.org/10.1093/imaman/dpn031.

29. Izady N, Worthington D. Setting staffing requirements for time dependent queueing networks: the case of accident and emergency departments. *Eur J Oper Res* 2012; 219: 531–40. https://doi.org/10.1016/j.ejor.2011.10.040.

30. Howick S, Ackermann F. Mixing OR methods *in practice*: past, present and future directions. *Eur J Oper Res* 2011; 215: 503–11. https://doi.org/10.1016/j.ejor.2011.03.013.

31. Brailsford SC, Eldabi T, Kunc M, Mustafee N, Osorio AF. Hybrid simulation modelling in operational research: a state-of-the-art review. *Eur J Oper Res* 2019; 278: 721–37. https://doi.org/10.1016/j.ejor.2018.10.025.

32. Viana J, Brailsford SC, Harindra V, Harper PR. Combining discrete-event simulation and system dynamics in a healthcare setting: a composite model for Chlamydia infection. *Eur J Oper Res* 2014; 237: 196–206. https://doi.org/10.1016/j.ejor.2014.02.052.

33. Pagel C, Banks V, Pope C, et al. Development, implementation and evaluation of a tool for forecasting short term demand for beds in an intensive care unit. *Oper Res Health Care* 2017; 15: 19–31. https://doi.org/10.1016/j.orhc.2017.08.003.

34. Harper PR, Pitt MA. On the challenges of healthcare modelling and a proposed project life cycle for successful implementation. *J Oper Res Soc* 2004; 55: 657–61. https://doi.org/10.1057/palgrave.jors.2601719.

35. Welch JD, Bailey NTJ. Appointment systems in hospital outpatient departments. *Lancet* 1952; 259: 1105–8. https://doi.org/10.1016/S0140-6736(52)90763-0.

36. Rosenhead J. Operational research in health services planning. *Eur J Oper Res* 1978; 2: 75–85. https://doi.org/10.1016/0377-2217(78)90103-0.

37. Flagle CD. Some Origins of operations research in the health services. *Oper Res* 2002; 50: 52–60. https://doi.org/10.1287/opre.50.1.52.17805.

38. The European Working Group on Operational Research Applied to Health Services. Past meetings. http://orahs.di.unito.it/meetings.html (accessed 14 February 2020).

39. The Institute for Operations Research and the Management Sciences. INFORMS Healthcare 2019: schedule. http://meetings2.informs.org/word press/healthcare2019/schedule (accessed 14 February 2020).

40. Brailsford S, Vissers J. OR in healthcare: a European perspective. *Eur J Oper Res* 2011; 212: 223–34. https://doi.org/10.1016/j.ejor.2010.10.026.

41. Monks T. Operational research as implementation science: definitions, challenges and research priorities. *Implement Sci* 2016; 11: 81. https://doi .org/10.1186/s13012-016-0444-0.

42. Pagel C, Zwart D. Wanted: talented, energetic, creative people to work on difficult, boring problems. No perks. *NEJM Catalyst* 2017; 3(6). https://catalyst .nejm.org/doi/full/10.1056/CAT.17.0341 (accessed 14 February 2020).

43. Craig P, Dieppe P, Macintyre S, et al. Developing and evaluating complex interventions: the new Medical Research Council guidance. *BMJ* 2008; 337: a1655. https://doi.org/10.1136/bmj.a1655.

44. Monks T, Pitt M, Stein K, James M. Maximizing the population benefit from thrombolysis in acute ischemic stroke. *Stroke* 2012; 43: 2706–11. https://doi.org/10.1161/STROKEAHA.112.663187.

45. Monks T, Pearson M, Pitt M, Stein K, James MA. Evaluating the impact of a simulation study in emergency stroke care. *Oper Res Health Care* 2015; 6: 40–9. https://doi.org/10.1016/j.orhc.2015.09.002.

46. Chalk D. Determining optimal locations for urgent care centres in Cornwall using computer modelling. *Br J Healthc Manag* 2019; 25: 235–40. https:// doi.org/10.12968/bjhc.2019.0034.

47. King M, Ramnarayan P, Seaton SE, Pagel C. Modelling the allocation of paediatric intensive care retrieval teams in England and Wales. *Arch Dis Child* 2019; 104: 962–6. http://dx.doi.org/10.1136/archdischild-2018-316056.

48. Eveborn P, Rönnqvist M, Einarsdóttir H, et al. Operations research improves quality and efficiency in home care. *Interfaces* 2009; 39: 18–34. https://doi.org/10.1287/inte.1080.0411.

49. Bowers J, Cheyne H, Mould G, et al. A multicriteria resource allocation model for the redesign of services following birth. *BMC Health Serv Res* 2018; 18: 656. https://doi.org/10.1186/s12913-018-3430-1.

50. Cribb A, Entwistle V, Mitchell P. Values and ethics. In: Dixon-Woods M, Brown K, Marjanovic S, et al., editors. *Elements of Improving Quality and Safety in Healthcare.* Cambridge: Cambridge University Press; forthcoming.

51. Institute of Medicine (US) Committee on Quality of Health Care in America. *Crossing the Quality Chasm: A New Health System for the 21st Century.* Washington, DC: National Academies Press; 2001. https://doi.org/10.17226/10027.

52. De Causmaecker P, Vanden Berghe G. A categorisation of nurse rostering problems. *J Sched* 2011; 14: 3–16. https://doi.org/10.1007/s10951-010-0211-z.

53. M'Hallah R, Alkhabbaz A. Scheduling of nurses: a case study of a Kuwaiti health care unit. *Oper Res Health Care* 2013; 2: 1–19. https://doi.org/10.1016/j.orhc.2013.03.003.

54. Drake RG. The nurse rostering problem: from operational research to organizational reality? *J Adv Nurs* 2014; 70: 800–10. https://doi.org/10.1111/jan.12238.

55. Kellogg D, Walczak S. Nurse scheduling: from academia to implementation or not? *Interfaces* 2007; 37: 355–69. https://doi.org/10.1287/inte.1070.0291.

56. Kunc M, Harper P, Katsikopoulos K. A review of implementation of behavioural aspects in the application of OR in healthcare. *J Oper Res Soc* 2020; 71: 1055–72. https://doi.org/10.1080/01605682.2018.1489355.

57. Pearson M, Monks T, Gibson A, et al. Involving patients and the public in healthcare operational research – the challenges and opportunities. *Oper Res Health Care* 2013; 2: 86–9. https://doi.org/10.1016/j.orhc.2013.09.001.

58. Robert G, Locock L, Williams O, et al. Co-producing and co-designing. In: Dixon-Woods M, Brown K, Marjanovic S, et al., editors. *Elements of Improving Quality and Safety in Healthcare.* Cambridge: Cambridge University Press; 2022. https://doi.org/10.1017/9781009237024.

59. Marshall M, Pagel C, French C, et al. Moving improvement research closer to practice: the researcher-in-residence model. *BMJ Qual Saf* 2014; 23: 801–5. http://dx.doi.org/10.1136/bmjqs-2013-002779.

60. Vindrola-Padros C, Pape T, Utley M, Fulop NJ. The role of embedded research in quality improvement: a narrative review. *BMJ Qual Saf* 2017; 26: 70–80. https://doi.org/10.1136/bmjqs-2015-004877.

61. Vindrola-Padros C, Eyre L, Baxter H, et al. Addressing the challenges of knowledge co-production in quality improvement: learning from the implementation of the researcher-in-residence model. *BMJ Qual Saf* 2019; 28: 67–73. https://doi.org/10.1136/bmjqs-2017-007127.

62. The Health Foundation. ABCi Mathematical Modelling and Analytics Academy. www.health.org.uk/improvement-projects/abci-mathematical-modelling-and-analytics-academy (accessed 15 February 2020).

63. MASHnet. The UK Network for Modelling & Simulation in Healthcare. https://mashnet.info/ (accessed 23 March 2022).

64. Hulshof PJH, Kortbeek N, Boucherie RJ, Hans EW, Bakker PJM. Taxonomic classification of planning decisions in health care: a structured review of the state of the art in OR/MS. *Health Syst* 2012; 1: 129–75. https://doi.org/10.1057/hs.2012.18.

65. Kirby MW. *Operational Research in War and Peace: The British Experience from the 1930s to 1970*. London: Imperial College Press; 2003. https://doi.org/10.1142/p247.

66. Winston WL, Goldberg JB. *Operations Research: Applications and Algorithms*. Belmont, CA: Brooks/Cole – Thomson Learning; 2004.

Cambridge Elements ☰

Improving Quality and Safety in Healthcare

Editors-in-Chief

Mary Dixon-Woods

THIS Institute (The Healthcare Improvement Studies Institute)

Mary is Director of THIS Institute and is the Health Foundation Professor of Healthcare Improvement Studies in the Department of Public Health and Primary Care at the University of Cambridge. Mary leads a programme of research focused on healthcare improvement, healthcare ethics, and methodological innovation in studying healthcare.

Graham Martin

THIS Institute (The Healthcare Improvement Studies Institute)

Graham is Director of Research at THIS Institute, leading applied research programmes and contributing to the institute's strategy and development. His research interests are in the organisation and delivery of healthcare, and particularly the role of professionals, managers, and patients and the public in efforts at organisational change.

Executive Editor

Katrina Brown

THIS Institute (The Healthcare Improvement Studies Institute)

Katrina is Communications Manager at THIS Institute, providing editorial expertise to maximise the impact of THIS Institute's research findings. She managed the project to produce the series.

Editorial Team

Sonja Marjanovic

RAND Europe

Sonja is Director of RAND Europe's healthcare innovation, industry, and policy research. Her work provides decision-makers with evidence and insights to support innovation and improvement in healthcare systems, and to support the translation of innovation into societal benefits for healthcare services and population health.

Tom Ling

RAND Europe

Tom is Head of Evaluation at RAND Europe and President of the European Evaluation Society, leading evaluations and applied research focused on the key challenges facing health services. His current health portfolio includes evaluations of the innovation landscape, quality improvement, communities of practice, patient flow, and service transformation.

Ellen Perry

THIS Institute (The Healthcare Improvement Studies Institute)

Ellen supported the production of the series during 2020–21.

About the Series

The past decade has seen enormous growth in both activity and research on improvement in healthcare. This series offers a comprehensive and authoritative set of overviews of the different improvement approaches available, exploring the thinking behind them, examining evidence for each approach, and identifying areas of debate.

Cambridge Elements ⹀

Improving Quality and Safety in Healthcare

Elements in the Series

Collaboration-Based Approaches
Graham Martin and Mary Dixon-Woods

Co-Producing and Co-Designing
Glenn Robert, Louise Locock, Oli Williams, Jocelyn Cornwell, Sara Donetto, and
Joanna Goodrich

The Positive Deviance Approach
Ruth Baxter and Rebecca Lawton

Implementation Science
Paul Wilson and Roman Kislov

Making Culture Change Happen
Russell Mannion

Operational Research Approaches
Martin Utley, Sonya Crowe, and Christina Pagel

A full series listing is available at: www.cambridge.org/IQ

Printed in the United States
by Baker & Taylor Publisher Services